Natural Relief from Arthritis

A Bio-Health Research Publication
by Dr Shaheen Perveen.

© 2006 Bio-Health Research Inc

You should consult your doctor/professional adviser before acting on any information contained in Natural Relief from Arthritis

Care and Cure for Arthritis

There's never been a more exciting time in the care and cure of arthritis. Medical miracles, innovation, progress, space age technology and treatments abound, amidst a plethora of wonder drugs. Today, relief is more readily available than ever before, as the basics of good health are being constantly rewritten as sufferers take treatment into their own hands. Old approaches are either making a serious comeback, or fading fast, to make room for scientific advances that continue to evolve. So what do we know about the disease that can help us to better treat it?

Arthritis has been with us since the advent of civilization. Neanderthal skeletons, Egyptian mummies and other ancient bones reveal a common disease - arthritis. One of the earliest written references to arthritis comes from the ancient Ayurvedic text – *Caraka Samhita* that describes the swollen, painful joints that commence with the hands and feet and gradually spreads to other parts of the body. Hippocrates mentioned it in his writings and it has been subsequently discussed through the centuries.

To stave off the painful malady, countless approaches were tried, one superseding the next in pursuit of more effective options. We've come a long way from decoctions of Peruvian bark, steel screws and plates to gold salt injections and finally today's living cartilage cell implants, joint fluid therapy and a variety of replacement surgeries.

Despite all round investigations and endless research, the etiology of arthritis remains a mystery. Besides injury, inheritance, infection, aging, obesity, abnormal metabolism and autoimmune reactions, there are hundreds of possible reasons attributed to this multifactorial disease. "Inflammation" is believed to be the most plausible cause that cuts across the entire spectrum of chronic diseases and plays a role in pathological conditions ranging from a simple allergy to more complex arthritis.

Simply put, inflammation is a perpetual orchestration of pro and anti inflammatory events in the body. The more inflammation you have, the faster the pace of acceleration towards chronic disease. We need to check inflammation in order to;
• Evade sudden death
• Suppress the immune system

• Control and manage arthritis, osteoporosis and related joint inflammation

The key to inflammation is maintaining the right balance – right hormonal balance, right pH (potential of Hydrogen) value, right ratio of fats, right co-ordination between Omega 3 and Omega 6, right proportion of protein and carbohydrates. Any mismatch or imbalance invites inflammation.

The Inflammation Factor

Inflammation is the body's fundamental way of protecting itself from injury, infection, or destruction of tissues. Think of it as immediate first aid, localized protective reaction, or the first line of defence that triggers a complex biological pathway of interrelated events. Inflammation can be said to be an ingenious adaptation, by which the body defends itself against clear and present danger.

A simple cut, wound, scrape, sunburn or even a mosquito bite is enough to provoke the body's inflammatory response to step in. The cellular mercenaries (composed of various white blood cells, plasma proteins, chemical messengers, etc.) arrive immediately and take control by resisting all the lurking bacteria, dirt, germs, foreign bodies, etc., and simultaneously initiate steps to repair the damaged tissue. This happens frequently, and is so intelligently handled by our natural in-built defense mechanism (inflammation) that, at times, we hardly notice or feel it. Moreover, inflammation is not confined to the skin but can occur internally as well. For instance, an upset stomach is inflammation caused by the body sensing food that it might be harmful to accept.

So far so good, and this is how inflammation works in a healthy human being. But ironically at times, the body's intelligent and sophisticated defence mechanism is thrown out of gear and inflammation actually harms and attacks the very tissues it is supposed to heal or repair.

The Chemistry of Inflammation

All animals are gifted with a microbial defence mechanism designed specifically to deal with injury and infection. It begins with acute phase response or in other words inflammation, which is a very complex cellular and molecular process.

The cellular components of the immune system – a variety of white blood cells - are prompt to recognize the disease-causing organism or the site of injury, and accordingly release the chemicals to initiate inflammation. This involves numerous cells, cell surface molecules, mediators and dozens of chemical messengers. Inflammatory chemicals cause blood vessels to dilate and leak. Plasma pours out in order to check the progress of the invading bacteria and simultaneously summons others immune defenders to join in.

Macrophages that float around in the blood stream are the first to spot any injury or infection, and they immediately release *cytokines* - chemicals (low molecule proteins) that carry messages between cells. One of the first cytokines to be released is known as *interleukin 1B*. It diffuses into tissues around the damaged cells and triggers a second wave of cytokines, which signal for further reinforcements. Immune cells like neutrophils, leukocytes, lymphocytes, follow and the site is flooded with various immune cells that trigger chain reactions in various ways.

Once these immune cells gain control over the situation, more macrophages arrive for the clean up process. They engulf the dead cells and this is the end of the inflammation process in a healthy person. Unfortunately, sometimes the story does not end here, and despite the elimination of the original trigger, these living soldiers or the macrophages keep releasing harmful neurotoxins and toxic radicals (oxygen free) and inflammation becomes self-perpetuating.

Signs and Symptoms of Inflammation

The underlying process for any type of inflammation is basically the same. The four basic physical signs identified with inflammation are – tumor, rubor, calor and dolor. This corresponds to swelling, pain, redness and heat.

• Swelling is the outcome of leaking plasma and arrival of immune cells at the required site of damage. The cells lining blood vessels allow the large protein molecules to leave the bloodstream and enter the inflamed tissue.

• Pain and inflammation go hand in hand. Pain is believed to result from chemical substances like serotonin or from tissue tension over the inflamed area. Pain occurs when the sensitive nerve endings become irritated and it serves as a warning that something is wrong in the body.

• Heat is detrimental to the growth of bacteria, which reproduce effectively at normal body temperature. Almost all injuries and infections cause fever, to check the growth of bacteria, sensitive to the slightest temperature increase. On the other hand, a raised body temperature accelerates the growth of the immune system and readies it for counterattack.

• Redness is a result of increase in local blood flow and to facilitate this process the blood vessels open to their widest diameter and make the vessel walls more permeable. Histamine, released by the special immune cell or mast cells, promotes greater blood flow so that more white blood cells can reach damaged or infected tissues.

Psychological symptoms include loss of energy or lethargy (due to fever/heat), loss of appetite, chills, headache, muscle stiffness and increased sensitivity to pain.

Chronic Inflammation

If all the 'on' and 'off' mechanism in acute inflammation process goes well, things return to normal with memories of temporary, minor discomfort and no permanent damage. In unhealthy conditions the inflammation process lingers and it passes on to a longer term 'chronic phase' – an example of inflammation gone awry. This broader implication is a matter for concern and was first observed by the cardiologists who noticed that besides cholesterol, chronic inflammation was also detrimental to the heart.

The scenario is like a body at war with itself. Heart, kidney, intestine - in fact any organ - can be the victim of inflammation as a part of autoimmune disorder. At times, there is no immediate risk of infection but still the immune system mistakenly triggers a low-grade inflammatory response, leading to cumulative damage and disease. Perhaps the most important inflammatory conditions to affect us are the various types of arthritis and rheumatism. Arthritis acquires different forms that produce inflammation of connective tissues, particularly the joints. Rheumatoid arthritis is another example of inflammation of the connective tissue where the inner linings or the synovial membranes are chronically inflamed.

Causes of Chronic Inflammation

As we age, there is an increase in level of pro-inflammatory (damaging) cytokines that contribute to the numerous inflammatory conditions. Moreover, aging weakens our ability to shut off the inflammatory process. Elderly people, who tend to be frail and inactive, exhibit more signs of inflammation than those who are young and active. Other factors include stress, toxins, insulin levels, obesity, etc.

The Key Agents of Inflammation

Food Matters

Choosing the right food is essential. What, how and when we eat offers some of the most potent, everyday remedies around us. Foods taken every day can treat and even cure inflammation and bolster our resistance to disease. With a little effort we can harness amazing therapeutic benefits from everyday food.

Foods containing arachidonic acid (eg. Eggs, organ meat, beef and dairy products) promote inflammation and so we can restrict their use. The body breaks down arachidonic acid into inflammatory compounds. We should give greater consideration to vegetables and fruits that have a low rating (60 or lower) on the glycemic index. This equates to food that is capable of calming and even reducing the inflammatory process.

Whole foods, cold water fish and extra virgin olive oil are welcome whereas processed foods, oils, animal fats, saturated fats, trans fats (hydrogenated) and margarine should be discouraged.

Undercooked food is neither desirable nor healthy but cooking at high temperatures is another risk factor leading to inflammation. Overcooked food (including so-called 'junk' foods like French fries, barbecued food, chips, fried foods, hamburgers and similar snacks) induce the formation of advanced glycation end (AGE) products or glycotoxins.

Glycation is an irreversible, destructive process (binding of protein molecule to glucose molecule) that occurs throughout the body. It changes the shape and properties of the protein structures which is rendered non functional and sets the body's alarm signal for the production of the damaging inflammatory cytokines. Glycation is implicated as a strong contributor to many progressive diseases of aging, like arterial stiffening, cataract etc.

The presence of glycotoxins in our living tissues (under the skin, arteries, eye lenses, joints, cartilage, etc.) increases the level of inflammatory cytokines. Depending on where AGES occur, it can lead to wrinkles, cataracts, arthritis, etc. which we commonly presume as a part of aging. Avoiding high temperature foods also keeps us free from carcinogens (the toxins related to gene-mutation) and other metabolic disorders.

Our diet can play a vital role in reducing or promoting inflammation. Simply eating too much is a factor that promotes the inflammatory response and suppresses the immune system. Besides choosing the right food, moderation is the key. Five to six smaller, nutritious and well-balanced meals spread throughout the day is considered to be healthier than fewer meals totalling the same quantity.

Different dietary fats have different effects on inflammation. Prostaglandins (one of the several chemicals that control inflammation) are made by the fats we eat. Choosing the right type of fat will create 'good' prostaglandins that will 'turn off' the inflammation in the body. Whereas 'bad' fats (margarines and cooking oils) will promote inflammation.

EPA or eicosapentaenoic acid (fat that is found in cold water fish, fish oils, Omega 3), alpha-linolenic acid (ALA, found in vegetables, beans, fruits and fish oil, flaxseed oil, wheat germ, walnut oils, etc.) and gamma-linolenic acid (GLA is found in Evening Primrose Oil, Hemp Oil, Borage Oil, etc.) are some of the healthy fats that do us good.

The Protein Pile-Up

Human proteins have now taken centre stage in medical research. More than 98% of diseases are related to problems with protein. The most direct information about any disease can be gleaned from the proteins. Molecules of protein are vital to the inflammation process. Coded as CD44, these protein molecules reside on the tip of the white blood cells and help the fighting process. However poor regulation of CD44 leads to the inflammatory diseases which provides the platform for cancer cells to break away from a primary tumor and circulate in the body.

The COX (cyclooxygenase) protein pathways are crucial mediators of inflammation. The body produces several forms of cyclooxygenase. COX1 and COX2 exist as two distinct but similar isozyms. The beneficial COX1 helps in blood clotting, pain and protection of stomach linings. The harmful COX2 that is present in the body only during inflammation, is an important link in the inflammation cascade. It inserts an oxygen molecule into arachidonic acid to synthesize prostaglandins, which are powerful triggers of pain and inflammation.

Prostaglandins are lipids (fatty substances) made from the fats that we eat. There are good and bad prostaglandins that promote or turn off inflammations. Fats from high fat meat and dairy products produce the unwelcome PG-2 in association with COX2, while fats from fish, Primrose, Flaxseed and Borage go into the making of healthy COX1. PG1 and PG3 in participation with COX1 exert anti-inflammatory effects and are healing in nature.

C-Reactive Protein (CRP) belongs to the pentraxin family of proteins, which is produced in the liver. It is released into the bloodstream during inflammation and these proteins latch onto the microbial invaders, marking them for destruction.

CRP measures inflammation and high levels (above 3 mg/L) of this protein increases the risk of heart attack and other diseases. The most common cause of an elevated level of CRP is infection and the levels fluctuate (from 3 mg to 1000 mg/L) from day to day which increases with age, smoking, blood pressure, fatigue, high protein diet, diabetes, depression, sleep disturbances and other factors.

Diseases Associated with Inflammation

Chronic inflammation is involved in diverse diseases. Seemingly unrelated, but these diseases have a common link – high levels of pro-inflammatory markers in their blood.

Some of these inflammatory conditions to affect us are allergy, Alzheimer's, anemia, arthritis (various conditions like rheumatoid arthritis, shoulder tendonitis or bursitis, gouty arthritis, polymyalgia rheumatica, etc), cancer, heart failure, fibromyalgia, fibrosis, kidney failure, lupus, pancreatitis, psoriasis, etc.

Medications For Inflammatory Diseases

Conventional Treatments

Medications available for treating inflammation, in fact, focus on treating pain. The painkillers are followed by non-steroidal anti-inflammatory drugs (NASAIDs) like ibuprofen, aspirin or naproxen. Most are purchased for easing arthritis more than for any other disorder.

NSAIDs have been with us for long and widely prescribed for the treatment of rheumatoid arthritis and osteoarthritis. They prevent inflammation by blocking the cyclooxygenase (COX) enzyme, which suppresses the synthesis of a hormonal substance called prostaglandins. This substance is also important in regulating how the kidneys excrete sodium and protein. If the drug is effective against arthritis, some effect on the kidney can't be ruled out. A fall in prostaglandin level invites gastric ulceration, renal insufficiency and prolonged bleeding time.

Blockage of the enzyme spells trouble for the stomach lining and it ends up with various adverse side effects, like water retention in the joint, which is one of the earliest signs that the cartilage in the joint is actually deteriorating. NSAIDs have been shown to cause devastating gastrointestinal damage. Prolonged use of NSAIDs may create holes in the stomach linings. In the US, more than 20,000 deaths occur due to long term use of NSAIDs and more than 100,000 people are hospitalized each year in the US as a result of adverse reactions from NSAIDs. Few of the NSAIDs like Oraflex and Zomax were removed from the market because of their association with fatalities.

In treating arthritis, NSAIDs prevent cartilage repair by slowing down the production of collagen and proteoglycans, while accelerating cartilage destruction. The higher the dosage and longer the usage the faster the destruction.

The new versions of NSAIDs that have appeared in the market are believed to be kinder to the stomach but may pose a potential risk to the heart. Aspirin may be hailed for its help in reducing heart attacks but its very strength exposes its greatest weakness. It inhibits clotting and so it also increases the risk of gastrointestinal bleeding, either from an ulcer or gastritis. It can also induce hemorrhagic stroke, caused by bleeding in the brain and tinnitus. Moreover, the required therapeutic dose (2-4 grams per day) is quite high and often results in toxicity.

COX2 inhibitors are marketed as 'painkillers with fewer gastrointestinal side effects' as compared to NASIDs. Celebrex and Vioxx became two of the most celebrated COX2 painkillers and were among the top ten selling drugs in the world, but neither has been found to be better at reducing pain than cheaper alternatives. Express Scripts released a study that 'the drugs are often prescribed unnecessarily, when a cheaper alternative would suffice.'

Natural Anti-inflammatory Options

Independently or in conjunction with your medications, there are some natural, nutritional supplements that do an excellent job of eliminating or limiting the inflammations. Moreover, unlike conventional remedies, they come without any fear or risk of side effects.

CELADRIN: In the long list of natural supplements Celadrin is a new entry with an impressive pedigree. It is the most effective natural anti-inflammatory compound prepared from a complex blend of esterified fatty acids and other active synergists. It provides fast acting (within 30 minutes) relief, which is rapid and deep enough to promote flexibility and healthy joint functions. Celadrin works by beneficially altering the body's production of chemical mediators that lead to inflammation and pain. Instead of focusing on symptoms, Celadrin addresses the cause and seeks remedial measures at the very core.

There is no known side effect or interaction with drugs or other natural pain relievers. By enhancing cell membranes, Celadrin enables the body to utilize other natural remedies more efficiently.

CURCUMIN: India has the lowest incidence of Alzheimer's anywhere in the world. This may be attributed to the everyday use of Turmeric. Ayurvedic practitioners have been using this medicinal rootstock since time immemorial. Besides dietary spice, it is used in the treatment of various illnesses, particularly as a topical treatment (in poultices) for treating inflamed joints. Curcumin – the polyphenolic pigments in the spice Turmeric that turns curry yellow is also a powerful anti-inflammatory antioxidant, which is stronger than hydrocortisone and its antioxidant action more active than Vitamin E. The possible anti-inflammatory activity of Curcumin includes inhibition of COX, LOX and other pro-inflammatory cytokines TNF, alpha and IL interleukin 1 Beta. Commission E approves Turmeric root for dyspeptic conditions.

BOSWELLIA: This gum resin has been popular since ancient times. Besides anti-inflammatory Boswellic acid, it contains various fatty acids. Boswellic acid and its various derivatives have anti-carcinogenic, anti-tumor and blood lipid lowering activities. Dried extracts are traditionally used to treat inflammatory conditions, particularly in osteoarthritis and rheumatoid arthritis, asthma and ulcerative colitis. It plays an active role in blocking the production of pro-inflammatory prostaglandins, 5-lipoxygenase chemicals and leukotriene synthesis. The gum resin is used as an ointment for sores and is a well-known household fumigant in some parts of the world (also referred to as Indian frankincense).

WHITE WILLOW BARK EXTRACT: Willow Bark has been with us since early use in ancient China, Greece and other parts of the world. It is mentioned in Dioscorides' *De Materia Medica* of the first century. Willow's anti-inflammatory action is attributed to salicylates present in the bark. It has the same effect on the body as aspirin (in fact, White Willow was the basis for the synthesis of aspirin) but with no side effects. The Commission E approves Willow Bark for diseases accompanied by fever, rheumatic ailments and headaches. The British Herbal Compendium indicates its use for rheumatic and arthritic conditions and feverish conditions such as influenza.

* According to a report published in *Rheumatology* (2001:40: 1388-93) an extract of Willow Tree Bark is as effective as a common prescription medication for the treatment of low back pain.

GINGER ROOT EXTRACT: Ginger has been used as a medicine and culinary herb since ancient times. It has remained a popular spice and medicinal plant in

India and China for thousands of years. Besides various other uses, Ginger's anti-inflammatory properties have long been used as a remedy for treating arthritis. It is also a strong antioxidant and an effective microbial agent for sores and wounds. Research suggests Ginger Root inhibits production of prostlandins and leukotrienes, which are involved in pain and inflammation. The Ginger rhizome contains a variety of chemicals like gingerol, zingerone and essential oils. Commission E approves the internal use of Ginger for dyspepsia and prevention of motion sickness.

* According to a study published in *OsteoArthritis and Cartilage* (2003: 11: 783-9), adults suffering from osteoarthritis of the knees may experience less pain and swelling and increased mobility in the knees by taking an extract of Ginger.

BROMELAIN: Bromelain, which is a phytonutrient derived from pineapple plant, is a group of proteolytic enzymes noted for its powerful anti-inflammatory actions. Usually large enzymes are broken down in the digestive tract but those in Bromelain are absorbed whole to a certain extent and this triggers systemic effects. Once in the blood, Bromelain reduces inflammation by thinning the blood and this affects the immune system.

Furthermore, it blocks the production of compounds that cause swelling and pain. It is known to reduce pain, swelling and inflammation associated with bruising, sprains, sports injuries, burns, wounds and arthritis. Commission E approves the use of Bromelain for acute post-operative and post-traumatic conditions of swelling.

* According to *Phytomedicine* (2002/ Dec), there is preliminary clinical evidence to support the contention that the anti-inflammatory and analgesic properties of Bromelain help to reduce symptoms of osteo and rheumatoid arthritis.

DEVIL'S CLAW: Devil's Claw is an African desert plant with tubers that contain a concentration of the compounds called iridoid glycosides (particularly harpagoside, which is gifted with anti inflammatory and pain killing actions), carbohydrates, phenols, amino acids and flavonoids. It is used as a herbal tea ingredient to treat back pain, painful, inflamed joints due to osteoarthritis and rheumatoid arthritis. It is also used as a tropical ointment to heal sores, boils and other skin problems. It also eases the stiffness of rheumatic diseases. Devil's Claw is approved by Commission E to restore appetite, dyspepsia, and degenerative disorders of the locomotor system.

* According to study published in *Phytomedicine* (2002: 9: 181-94), a standardized extract of the herb Devil's Claw is effective for the majority of people with low back, knee, or hip pain.

OLIVE OIL: The Mediterranean diet is appreciated for its 'olive oil' content linked to reduced risk of heart disease. FDA now allows this vital health claim to appear on packaging labels on olive oils and foods made with olive oil. Besides benefits to the heart, olive oil is equally helpful in reducing the inflammation associated with rheumatoid arthritis. The health benefits of olive oil come from its antioxidants – including Vitamin E – and its principle monounsaturated fat, oleic acid, which is an Omega-9 fatty acid. Oleocanthol – the substance isolated from extra-virgin olive oil, inhibits two enzymes involved in the process of inflammation (COX1 and COX2).

* According to *Nature* (2005:437:45-6), a substance found in extra-virgin olive oil has anti-inflammatory effects similar to those of ibuprofen (Mortin, Advil).

CHONDROTIN SULPHATE: Belonging to the family of GAGs (glycosaminoglycans), chondrotin sulphate is a complex protein molecule – sort of membrane fluidizer that provides elasticity and protection to the bones. Found in cartilages of most mammals and also in bone, cornea, skin and the arterial wall, it provides cartilage with structure, holding water and nutrients that allows other molecules to move through cartilage. Depletion of Chondrotin Sulphate erodes the cartilage, leading to pain and inflammation. Supplements help to maintain the healthy joints and cartilage.

* According to a study in *OsteoArthritis and Cartilage* (2004: 12: 269-76), people who experience pain and poor joint function in the knees due to osteoarthritis may reduce symptoms by intermittently taking oral Chondrotin Sulphate.

GLUCOSAMINE SULPHATE: Found naturally in the body by the combination of the simple sugar glucose with the amino acid glutamine. Glucosamine Sulphate is vital for the production and repair of new cartilage and synthesis of synovial fluid. It outperforms other anti-inflammatory drugs and within a short period of time, Glucosamine Sulphate supplement boosts regeneration of cartilage, enhances the production of your joint's oils (synovial fluid), improves the pain, inflammation and stiffness of rheumatism and arthritis. The best thing about Glucosamine Sulphate is that despite long-term use, there are 'no harmful side effects' and it complements other supplements.

FISH OILS: People still believe that the fish oils (eicosapentaenoic acid or EPA and docosahexaenoic acid or DHA) literally 'oil' the joints and relieve the pain and stiffness associated with ageing and arthritis. Rheumatoid arthritis is a systemic inflammatory disease that presents an abnormal fatty acid profile, which is deficient in essential fatty acids. RA is also believed to be the outcome of oxidative stress which involves an excess release of pro-inflammatory compounds like tumor necrosis factor – *alpha* and *interleukin 1beta* in the body. Now science is beginning to show that saturated fats from animal foods promote inflammation but fats from fish oil are beneficial in alleviating the symptoms of several inflammatory diseases. Precisely, it is the eicosapentaenoic acid or EPA content in fish oil that offers the protective benefit.

* According to a study published in *Nutrition* (2005: 21:131-6) people with rheumatoid arthritis can reduce their symptoms by supplementing with fish oil, and supplementing with olive oil can add to the benefit.

* According to *The Journal of Rheumatology* (2004: 31: 1551-6) supplementing with fish oil may decrease the symptoms of systemic lupus erythematosus.

* According to *Rheumatology International* (2002: 23: 27-36) anti-inflammatory diet and fish oil supplements are both helpful for people with rheumatoid arthritis, but combining them has an even greater effect.

GAMMA-LINOLENIC ACID (GLA): Gamma-linolenic acid is an essential fatty acid like the EPA and DHA found in fish oil. It is metabolized in the body to form prostaglandins which play a major role in mediating inflammation, blood clotting and are involved in the immune response against infections. GLA is found naturally to varying extents in the fatty acid fraction of some plant seed oils like Evening Primrose Seed Oil (7-14% of total fatty acids), in Borage Seed Oil (20-27%) and in Blackcurrant Seed Oil (15-20%). GLA has anti-inflammatory and anti-thrombotic actions. GLA supplied in the form of Evening Primrose Oil or Borage Seed Oil has been studied for its positive effects in arthritis and other inflammatory process. GLA is also useful in other rheumatological disorders.

GREEN LIPPED MUSSELS: Green Lipped Mussel extract from New Zealand has been shown to be useful in promoting healthy joint function, particularly in rheumatoid arthritis and osteoarthritis. Research primarily focuses on OA and RA, and these extracts significantly reduce pain and stiffness of the joints. Glycoproteins in the Green Lipped Mussel are believed to check inflammation in arthritic joints by preventing the white blood cells from moving into the joints. One animal study even found this mussel extract to significantly reduce stomach ulcers resulting from taking NSAIDs.

The Celadrin Scenario

Celadrin is the most highly praised among the long list of natural anti-inflammatory products. It is fast achieving star status as compelling evidence emerges of its widespread benefits and a growing body of research seems to support Celadrin as the best contemporary available option.

Celadrin works faster than all other natural remedies. Imagine as little as thirty minutes to begin cumulative relief from pain and restoration of mobility. Unlike a host of alternatives that do offer visible relief but simultaneously unfurl a chain of potentially fatal side effects, Celadrin's safety profile is impeccable. It is safe and non-toxic even at higher doses.

What is Celadrin?

Celadrin is a genuine breakthrough that heralds care and comfort for the unhealthy joints. It is the latest, most effective and natural anti-inflammatory product that restores flexibility and eases aching, painful joints, muscles and tissues in a very short time. Besides being fast, Celadrin assures optimal joint health that functions on a cumulative basis with no reported side effects.

Celadrin is available as tablet, capsule, soft gel and cream. Both oral and topical applications were shown to be equally effective with 95.1% absorption rate.

Celadrin's Composition

Celadrin is made from a patented complex blend of esterified fatty acid carbons, derived from bovine tallow oil and olive oil, besides other active synergists. The esterifying process makes the fatty acids stable so that it does not react with oxygen. Celadrin is scientifically designed so that the proprietary compounds are rapidly absorbed and proffer instant and continuous relief. With Celadrin one is better off tomorrow and the next day – it just gets better every day!

Celadrin's Modus Operandi

Ccladrin operates quite similarly to, but much more effectively than, the essential fatty acids (EPA and DHA) from fish oil.

• Fish oil lipids alter the fat content of the membrane phospholipids and hinder the production of eicosanoids that mediate inflammation. Fatty acids from the fish oils reduce cytokine synthesis and suppress cell activation.

• Fatty acids in olive oil have been shown to inhibit endothelial (the thin cells that line the inside of the various body cavities) activation and to reduce tissue responsiveness to cytokines.

• Fatty acids in Celadrin inhibit inflammation in endothelial cells and decrease pro-inflammatory effects of arachidonic and other fatty acids.

• Celadrin tends to reduce the production of the negative immune factor (IL-6) and the control of the immune factors responsible for inflammation.

• Celadrin lubricates the cell membranes throughout the body.

Celadrin at the Cellular Level

Celadrin dives down to the biological core of life. Down to the level of cell and more precisely the cell membrane, which is the organized structure that separates and shields the cell from its neighbouring cells and the outside world. A major component of the cell membrane is the structural lipid molecule that makes up the bulk of the cell membrane's surface area. The cell membrane is akin to a border, as well as a wall, which plays a crucial role by regulating the nutrients, minerals and electrolytes, drugs and other compounds. The membrane decides what should remain inside and outside the cell. This is always changing and the lipids help to regulate this traffic. There are several hundred types of lipid attached to the membrane of a single living cell.

Celadrin's composition is in close harmony with the cell membrane's consistency which is akin to olive oil and the inner layer of the lipids contain more unsaturated fatty acid chains. Celadrin ensures a healthy environment at the cellular level by enhancing the cell's integrity and functioning. The cells are continuously exposed to body stressors that impair and impede the membrane's lipid peak performance. The damage culminates in cellular short circuit, leading to the demise of the cell, which ultimately triggers pain and inflammation. Celadrin's unique composition rescues the cells by enhancing the lipid structure of the cell membrane. This makes the cells healthy and more energized which can now repair and regenerate faster, besides being ready for optimum, all round performance.

The Science behind Celadrin
Celadrin has been clinically studied at various stages with results appearing in numerous peer publications including Journal of Rheumatology and Journal of Strength and Conditioning Research.

For oral application, Celadrin was studied using a double blind, multi-centre, placebo-controlled trial (the most scientifically validated type) that assessed for the range of motion, pain levels, timed up and go from a chair, timed stair climbing and endurance test. 64 participants in the age group 37 to 77 were given Celadrin capsules and were evaluated at the beginning of the trial, after 30 days and at the end of the study after 68 days. Compared to the placebo group, those who were given Celadrin exhibited greater flexibility, fewer pains and were able to walk greater distances.

For topical application of Celadrin cream, the study involved 42 patients with osteoarthritis of the knee. Participants were either given a placebo or Celadrin cream. Patients were evaluated after 30 minutes and then at the conclusion of the trial after 30 days. Those who received Celadrin reported reduced pain and stiffness, improved balance and strength and greater flexibility. All patients using Celdarin cream reported significant improvement in their conditions as compared to the patients on the placebo. The initial observation after 30 minutes of application showed exciting results of all round relief.

Celadrin compared to other Joint Health Products
COX2 inhibitors are shadowed with numerous side effects. There are serious doubts about their safety

profile. In April 2002, FDA announced that Vioxx would require new information on its label noting that it might be linked to an increased risk of heart attack and high blood pressure. *Journal of Bone and Mineral Research* (May 2002) revealed that COX2s may impair healing of bone fractures.

Besides side effects, the pain relief offered by COX2 inhibitors is short lived. Celadrin is precisely focused on cause and relief comes from the chemistry of cells. The cells (membranes and lipids) are restored and optimized to good health, which leads to healthy joints and freedom from inflammation and pain. Moreover, Celadrin is faster with benefits that are cumulative and free from side effects.

Compared to Glucosamine, Chondrotin Sulphate, SAMe and other natural supplements, Celadrin's beneficial effects have been proven far superior and much faster. Celadrin provides relief and restoration of a wide range of joint health conditions and inflammations that include sports injuries, osteoarthritis, rheumatoid arthritis, fibromyalgia, gout, lupus, bursitis, tendonitis and various others conditions.

The Healthy Joint

The development of joints is valued as the most stunning evolutional feat. They have evolved in a unique way and are designed to permit either a lot or very little movement. Gifted with 143 joints and 206 bones (one quarter of the bones in an adult skeleton are located in the feet), we can perform an infinite variety of movements with remarkable fluidity and flexibility.

Consider the most free moving hip joint (ball and socket type) that performs the most flexible range of movements which can swing in almost any direction. Hinge joints perform limited movements in only one direction like those of the fingers, elbow, toes and knees. Life without the saddle joint in the thumb would be hard to imagine. Picking up a pin or tiny objects would be difficult in the absence of this precious joint.

In an average lifetime, a person flexes his finger joints over twenty-five million times! When we walk, the thigh bone (longest bone in the body) is capable of bearing a pressure of 1200lbs per square inch. Some of the joints support the equivalent of six times our body weight.

Between the bones lies a rubbery, pliable cartilage pad which serves as a protective cushion or shock absorber that allows the ends of the bones to move against each other almost without friction. The joint is capable of withstanding enormous pressure and in so doing, it slowly releases water from the cartilage. Maintaining this precious cartilage is the key to keeping joint problems in control.

A cartilage is a unique, resilient, living tissue that is continually broken down and replaced. It is made up of 70-80% water (that gives the cartilage its sponge-like quality) and the rest is made up of two vital compounds – collagen fibres (made out of hydrolyzed amino aids from protein) and proteoglycans (big molecules made up of sugar and proteins). Collagen fibres impart elasticity, give the cartilage its shock absorbing properties and are a key building block for several overall processes of the body. Proteoglycans respond to our movements by helping the cartilage to stretch and then bounce back when we move.

Between the bones is a joint cavity, which is enclosed by a flexible capsule that guards the joints against dislocation. The inner lining of the capsule is marked by a membrane called synovium, which produces a thick synovial fluid that nourishes and lubricates the space between the cartilage covered, joint-forming bones. Just outside the capsule lies the thick strong bands or ligaments, which help the bone, remain firm. The cartilage receives its nutrients by diffusion from the synovial fluid and from the bone. Joint function depends largely on the health of the cartilage in the joint and the synovial membrane. In the absence of healthy cartilage that cushions the bone, severe pain is experienced when the bones rub against each other.

The joints become more prone to damage as we age. The water content diminishes and the ability of cartilage decreases. Injury or inflammation or too much stress can further damage the cartilage leading to osteoarthritis.

This damage to the joint comes without any obvious signals or warning pain because the cartilage is not linked by nerves. By the time we get signals of pain, discomfort and disability, a significant amount of injury may have already occurred. Moreover, it can be confused with joint pain, which may in fact be sore muscles or tendons in the area. Arthritis related pains are persistent and often accompanied with stiffness and swollen joints. Normal muscle pains or any other kind of discomfort around the joint should vanish within a day or two. If the pain lingers for no obvious reasons, it could possibly be the beginning of arthritis and one should consult a doctor. The diversity of the forms of arthritis and rheumatism is further compounded by various stages of the disease. Happily, medical advances mean that for almost all forms and stages of joint trouble there is considerable relief available, if not a total cure.

EXERCISE – The Arthritis Therapy

Besides a nutritional supplement and low fat diet, some exercise benefits those suffering from arthritis. Once it was believed that exercise was not advisable, as it would damage your joints. Today, people praise and appreciate exercise as a vital – even joyful – part of life and living with arthritis. Exercises like swimming, stretching or simply walking helps to reduce joint pain and stiffness, build strong muscles around the joints, and increase flexibility and endurance. Fibromyalgia patients are particularly advised to get regular aerobic exercise such as walking and cycling along with stretching to prevent muscle spasms.

Lack of physical activity or exercise is believed to be the prime reason for worsening of the disability among elderly people with arthritis. This can be countered with regular, and modest to vigorous, physical activity. Ancient Chinese meditative art or *Tai Chi* has turned out to be a powerful tool for the elderly. With features like slow and graceful movements, the traditional Chinese art is becoming an accessible and fashionable choice for sufferers.

* According to the *American Journal of Clinical Nutrition* (2005:82:451-5), Eating cartenoid rich foods may help protect against inflammatory polyarthritis (inflammation of two or more joints), most commonly a manifestation of rheumatoid arthritis).

* According to *Arthritis and Rheumatism* (2005:52:1274-82), Regular vigorous physical activity can preserve functioning – such as the ability to work, dress, shop, and cook – that is often impaired in many older people with arthritis.

Arthritis Today

Arthritis is one of the most prevalent chronic health problems. Arthritis is defined as inflammation of one or more joints, which result in pain, swelling and limited movement. It is a complex disorder that encompasses over 100 distinct conditions. Nearly 1 in 3 adults in the US suffer from arthritis. 15% of the population in the UK has long-term, arthritis-related problems.

Something common to these 100 plus conditions is that they all affect the musculoskeletal system and particularly the joints. Arthritis rarely kills, but certainly painful movements, swollen joints, morning stiffness and at times disfigured joints can bring life to a screeching standstill. Certain conditions may interfere with the functioning of the other parts of the body like the bones, muscles and even internal organs, which can lead to further complications.

Arthritis is no longer a disease purely associated with old folks as it can affect anyone, irrespective of age and this includes children as well. The reason behind arthritis and related articular diseases is unknown but there are plenty of hypotheses. If left untreated, it can flare up with serious implications.

Osteoarthritis

Of more than over hundred different types of arthritis, osteoarthritis (OA) is the most common and possibly the oldest. It is also called 'wear and tear' arthritis, which is associated with age. As we grow old, it is likely that we may experience some degree of primary arthritis.

Secondary osteoarthritis is a condition with an apparent cause (like injury, obesity, hereditary, etc.) that leads to the breakdown of the cartilage.

In joints with OA, the cartilage that cushions bones where they meet becomes damaged and worn over the years which leads to pain, swelling and stiffness of the joints. This can affect any joint but the most likely victims are knee, finger joints, spine and hip joints. OA of the knee is the most common and in the very worst cases, bones begin to come in contact with each other.

The breakdown of the articular cartilage is attributed to a combination of mechanical, bio-chemical and genetic factors. The chemical factor is attributed to the poor supply of choncdrocytes, which leads to insufficient collagen and proteoglycans, which are vital to healthy joints. These chondrocytes are equally capable of repairing the damaged cartilages.

The earliest symptom of OA is pain, which stems from the inflammation of the joint lining or is the outcome of deterioration of healthy cartilage. The pain indicates the amount of injury that has occurred. As the cartilage begins to wear out, the bones rub against each other resulting in pain, loss of mobility, deformity and dysfunction. The damage spreads, which causes more pain, inflammation and stiffness.

A joint affected by osteoarthritis tries to repair itself and the tissues surrounding the joint becomes active. At times this internal healing process (mostly in small finger joints) is so successful that we may not experience the pain. Some people may not even realize that they are suffering from osteoarthritis. However the repair is not always successful (as in large joints) and certainly very slow, and at times, it culminates in more severe osteoarthritis. As part of the healing process, synovium becomes overactive and produces extra fluid, which in fact builds up in the joint space and simply aggravates the situation.

If osteoarthritis is left untreated, the cartilage will deteriorate further and result in debilitating pain. It may even end up in deformity (though uncommon) due to loss of cartilage, wear and tear of bones and the growth of bony edges (osteophytes or bony spurs).

Further complications arise when calcification or chondrocalcinosis sets in. In this stage chalky deposits (calcium crystals) develop in the cartilage and they disband themselves to irritate the synovium, which makes the joint hot, red and swollen.

WHAT CAUSES OSTEOARTHRITIS?

The possible causes of osteoarthritis can be summed up as the outcome of injury, stress on joints and the aging process. A major injury, fracture or operation on a joint can reveal itself as osteoarthritis later in life. At times osteoarthritis pains are linked to unusual stress, over use or injury to the joints.

Overweight people are prone to osteoarthritis. The extra weight adds up to the discomfort and trouble for the joints. The knees, hips, finger joints, thumb joints and lower spine are most affected in OA. Being overweight increases the risk of osteoarthritis, which is more common in men up to the age of 55. Beyond that age it becomes more common in women. Wearing high heels or poor posture adds to the burden on the joints and women become at greater risk of osteoarthritis.

At times the nature of a job like repetitive bending, kneeling, squatting or any superfluous exercise may be the crucial factor related to osteoarthritis.

SYMPTOMS & SIGNS OF OSTEOARTHRITIS

Initially, osteoarthritis begins with pain and stiffness that remains confined to one or few joints. The stiffness tends to be worse in the morning but gradually loosens up. The pain worsens with exertion, exercise or repetitive use and by the end of the day the pain is more evident. Rest brings relief but as the disease progresses pain maybe more intense and linger even when resting. Usually the knee, hip, hands or spine are affected but at times, wrists, elbows and ankles can be sites of osteoarthritis.

The joint may not move freely and at times it may appear swollen due to extra accumulation of the synovial fluid or the growth of osteophytes. However, large joints swellings are unusual in OA.

As the years go by, osteoarthritis (if left untreated) gets worse and may become more painful and disabling. However, most osteoarthritis sufferers are not severely disabled by it and even the level of pain may become static.

X-ray exposes osteoarthritis even if there is no pain. Sometimes, one may have severe symptoms but only minor changes are evident by X-ray. Osteophytes and choncdrocalcinosis that appear relatively late in the disease are easily identified in X-rays. Chondrocalcinosis mainly occurs in the knee joint of the elderly and at times these calcium crystals result in very painful swellings.

* According to the *Journal of Rheumatalogy* (2002:29:1708-12), CFA (Celadrin) provides an improvement in knee range of motion and overall function in patients with OA of the knee. CFA (Celadrin) may be an alternative to the use of NSAID drugs for the treatment of OA.

* According to *Phytomedicine* (2004:11:567-75), taking a soy protein supplement might reduce men's pain and disability from osteoarthritis.

Rheumatoid Arthritis

Unlike osteoarthritis that remains confined to a few joints with disrupted cartilages, rheumatoid arthritis (RA) is a chronic inflammatory illness that involves not only the multiple joints like fingers, wrist and legs but other connective tissue as well. RA is an autoimmune disease characterized by an overactive immune system that turns its attack to body tissues instead of invading pathogens.

In rheumatoid arthritis the chronic inflammation originates in the lining of the joints and causes pain, swelling, stiffness and may even lead to the loss of function in the joints. Rheumatoid arthritis is a progressive, systemic and symmetric disease, which means it affects the entire body and usually involves the same joints on both sides.

In the second stage the cells divide and grow rapidly, which causes the lining (synovium) to thicken. This is followed by the final stage where the inflamed cells release enzymes that may even digest the bone and cartilage, which in turn often causes the joint to loose its shape and alignment leading to loss of movement and further pain.

In rheumatoid arthritis inflammation takes place within the synovium. The joint appears swollen and red due to the increase in flow of blood. The swelling is due to the build up of extra fluid and cells in the synovium. The swelling triggers pain due to the stretching of the capsule, followed by the irritation of the nerve endings.

Rheumatoid arthritis usually first appears between the ages of 25 and 50 but it may strike at any age and even target children.

WHAT CAUSES RHEUMATOID ARTHRITIS?

RF or rheumatoid factor is a special antibody that is active against normal antibodies present in the bloodstream. RF factor is not directly responsible for the inflammatory process but simply acts as a marker for the disease. Precise causes underlying rheumatoid arthritis are unknown but it is believed to be an autoimmune, multifactorial disorder with genetic predisposition.

In rheumatoid arthritis inflammation, T-cells become overactive and invite B-cells to attack the body's own tissues. The T-cells further alert the leukocytes which get into action by inviting more white blood cells to the site. This prompts more blood to flow to the joint. This internal strife results in damaged cartilage, ligaments and sometimes even bones.

SYMPTOMS & SIGNS OF RHEUMATOID ARTHRITIS

Inflamed joints appear warm to touch, tender, swollen, red and show reduced motion. The symptoms are unpredictable in rheumatoid arthritis and often appear for the first time after a bout of severe stress (something like death, divorce, loss, etc.) or injury or change of environment.

In RA the disease progresses very slowly and usually begins with finger joints, which become swollen. However, in a few cases rheumatoid arthritis spreads very rapidly. These joints may appear stiff in the morning or after a period of rest. Muscles attached to the affected joints may lose strength.

Pain and swelling of the joints may appear intermittently. The severity may vary and at times it may create an impression of wellbeing with the fading of symptoms like pain and swelling. During flare-ups the symptoms return and often there is a period of relative remission. Beyond the joints, rheumatoid arthritis can inflame the salivary glands, tear glands, (dry eyes or lesions of the eye may occur), lungs, heart and even the blood vessels.

ESR levels are revealed through blood tests, which indicates the presence of an inflammatory process in the body. People with an increased amount of ESR may have rheumatoid arthritis. Blood tests can further detect the presence of an abnormal antibody - rheumatoid factor. Presence of RF is not a sure sign that a person is suffering from rheumatoid arthritis. Onset of RA usually occurs between the ages of 30 and 50 but it can strike suddenly at any time in life, including in childhood.

* According to a study published in *Nutrition* (2005: 21:131-6), people with rheumatoid arthritis can reduce their symptoms by supplementing with fish oil, and supplementing with olive oil can add to the benefit.

* According to *Annals of Rheumatic Diseases* (2003: 62: 208-14), people suffering from rheumatoid arthritis (RA) may experience decreased inflammation in their joints, improved physical function, and increased vitality by consuming a Mediterranean diet.

* According to *Rheumatology* (2001:40: 1175-9), a strict vegetarian diet led to improvement in symptoms of rheumatoid arthritis (RA).

Fibromyalgia

Linked to chronic muscle and joint pain, Fibromyalgia is severe enough to disrupt patients' lives. Surprisingly, diagnostic tests reveal no signs of joint abnormalities or muscle damage. It is referred to as a hidden, systemic disorder and may appear independently or accompanied with other forms of arthritis. This peculiar syndrome is characterized by generalized pain, besides symptoms like depression, chronic fatigue, headache and memory impairment.

Fibromyalgia mostly affects women aged 25 to 55 and ranks next only to osteoarthritis, as the most common disorder characterized by wide spread musculoskeletal pain, debilitating fatigue, stiffness, multiple tender points, sleep disorder, depression and cognitive difficulties.

In the absence of any outward sign, it is difficult to locate fibromyalgia, for which there is no specific test like an X-ray, blood tests, scans, etc. Doctors go by the tender point exam to ascertain this disorder, which reluctantly gained acceptance from the medical fraternity. It was not until 1987 that fibromyalgia was recognized as a true illness. It is all about pain and uneasiness from within but unlike arthritis, fibromyalgia does not cause permanent damage or disability but simply lingers for a long time.

18 tender points have been identified between the base of the skull and the knees. They reflect the tenderness that occurs in specific localized areas. These points occur in pairs on various parts of the body and the pain appears to be well distributed on both sides of the neck, spine, shoulders and hips. These tender points are painful when pressed.

WHAT CAUSES FIBROMYALGIA?

Fibromyalgia is elusive. Several symptoms of fibromyalgia are almost identical to that of other types of arthritis. Fibromyalgia is believed to be the outcome of injury, trauma or prolonged illness that has affected the central nervous system.

1. Defective muscle metabolism could be the reason for fibromyalgia. Poor flow of blood diminishes the muscular power which is believed to trigger fatigue and fibromyalgia.
2. Physiological abnormality by way of genetic predisposition is another possibility, which may flare up in conjunction with viral or bacterial infection.

3. Loss of estrogen (menopause) has been suggested as another plausible cause for fibromyalgia as it is more common among women in the age group of 40 to 55. Moreover, during menopause hormonal changes take over and this is a likely cause for depression.

4. Low levels of serotonin (magnesium) in people with fibromyalgia explain why they experience such an abnormally high level of pain and lack of deep sleep. Serotonin tones down the severity of pain signals and it is believed to regulate sleep, mood, appetite and sexual desires.

5. Prolonged stress and depression are closely linked to fibromyalgia. In both the situations brain chemistry is altered and the brain produces substances like neuropeptides and hormones that are more sensitive to pain and this leads to fibromyalgia.

SYMPTOMS & SIGNS OF FIBROMYALGIA

Fibromyalgia symptoms and its severity vary from person to person. Deep muscular pain, chronic fatigue and sleep disorder are usually the most prominent symptoms of fibromyalgia. People with fibromyalgia rarely reach the coveted delta sleep or the deep, restorative sleep.

* According to Arthritis and *Rheumatism* (2004:51:890-8), exercise leads to improvements in mood, ability to function, and overall symptoms in people with fibromyalgia.

Gout

Gout is one of the most common forms of arthritis characterized by sudden, severe attacks of pain, redness and tenderness of joints. This complex disorder appears suddenly, usually at night and without any warning. It can affect anyone but men are more susceptible than women, who are affected only after menopause.

Gout usually affects only one or two joints at a time. Most often it is the feet, ankle or the large joint of the big toe but it can occur in your knees, hands and wrists as well. Within 12-24 hours swelling in the affected joint, which turns red and shiny, follows pain. The pain ceases after five to ten days and the discomfort gradually diminishes over the week, leaving behind a normal joint. There may be intervals of many months and even years before gout reappears.

The inflammation in the joint is attributed to the build up of uric acid, which is supposed to dissolve in the blood. It is a metabolic disease and part of normal breaking down and building of food and body tissues. Too much of this acid results in sedimentation in the joints or the surrounding tissue that sparks pain, inflammation and swelling. Either there is too much uric acid or the process of elimination is very poor which results in accumulation of these needle-like crystals (urate) that trigger pain, swelling and inflammation.

Higher than normal levels of uric acid can be due to genetic inheritance, obesity or high alcohol intake, medication for blood pressure or high intake of food rich in purines (substances found in food that produce a lot of uric acid).

Treatment of gout lies in reduction of purines (liver, kidney, sweetbreads, red meat, shellfish, scallops, peas, lentils, beans and alcohol), revision of drugs to cure blood pressure, higher intake of water. According to new research holding ice packs on the afflicted joint does ease the pain of a gout attack. The misconception is that cooling the joints may promote crystal formation.

Systemic Lupus Erythematosus

Systemic Lupus Erythematosus is a disease in which a person's immune system attacks its own organs and tissues. It is also a multisystem disease as it can affect many different tissues and organs in the body like the joints, skin, kidney, lungs, nervous system, blood cells, heart and lungs. It affects 10 times as many women as men. Though lupus is a chronic disease, it is characterized by periods when the disease activity is minimal or almost absent followed by period of activity or relapse. It is also referred to as a "great imitator' because its symptoms are so varied that it is often confused with other disorders.

Lupus is an autoimmune disease that triggers inflammation with factors that remain unexplained but hereditary or genetic links, environmental pollution like silica dust or ultraviolet rays, mismatch of medications are believed to be the possible reasons that may trigger lupus. Research also suggests that it may originate in the biological process of clearing old and damaged cells from the body.

At the onset, the manifest symptoms are fatigue, fever and muscle and joint pain – a flu-like syndrome. The arthritis of lupus is normally found on both sides of the body and does not cause damage to the joints. The most affected joints are hands, knees and wrist. In more than half of all people with lupus, kidney and lung (chest pain while deep breathing) are involved. Diagnosis of lupus can be suspected by symptoms but it can only be confirmed by blood tests.

Management of lupus depends on symptoms and their severity.

Bursitis

Bursitis is the inflammation of the bursa, which is a small fluid filled sack that cushions the area of friction between tendon and bone or skin. These little sacks are lined with synovial cells, which secrete a fluid (akin to a lubricant that is rich in collagen and proteins) when parts of the body move. Most people have around 160 bursae throughout the body. This is intended to reduce friction between moving parts of the body like shoulder, elbow, knee, hip and heel. When this lubricating fluid becomes infected (by bacteria) or gets overworked with too much action or movement, the painful inflammation is referred to as bursitis.

Usually bursitis affects the areas surrounding the joints in your shoulder, elbow or hips. Pain associated with bursitis usually vanishes within a week if cared for and treated properly but flare-ups of bursitis can be frustrating.

The inflamed bursa can be identified by dull ache or stiffness in the infected part. The pain in the region worsens with movement or pressure, it appears swollen or warm and the skin may show redness. Bursitis of the hip does not display any visible symptom of swelling or redness due to the location of bursae.

Trauma, infection and crystal deposits are few of the common causes of bursitis. Trauma causes inflammatory bursitis from repetitive injury acquired through sports or occupational activities. This results in the widening of the blood vessels, which allows the protein and extra cellular fluids into the bursae, which react by becoming swollen.

Bursae are prone to infections, particularly the ones that are close to the surface of the skin. Most of this type of septic bursitis occurs in men. Diseases like gout or rheumatoid arthritis may lead to bursitis with crystal deposits. Uric acid, a byproduct of daily metabolism does not break down in conditions like gout and so this acid crystallizes and deposits in the joints.

Rest, application of ice, immobilization of the affected area, physical therapy and minor medication are some of the simple treatments that go with bursitis, which normally disappears within a week or two. In the case of infection, antibiotics may be prescribed. Instead of NSAIDS, the better and safer option can be prescribed as Celadrin cream for local application and the corresponding Celadrin tablet or capsules.

Tendonitis

Tendonitis is an inflammation of the tendon - end parts of the thick and tough fibrous cords that attach muscles to bone. Usually the pain and tenderness is most common around the shoulders, elbows and knees but can also occur in hips, heels and wrists.

Tendonitis is identified by pain and tenderness and at times a mild swelling which may result from occupational activities, repetitive or forceful motions, continued stress on the muscles, over use of the muscles during play or work or simple injury that can damage or tear the sheath of tissue surrounding the tendon. The damage can also be attributed to wear and tear due to aging or as an outcome of any systemic inflammation linked to rheumatoid arthritis.

A severe rupture of the tendon may invite surgical attention but usually relief comes from rest, application of ice and medications that reduce the pain and inflammation of tendonitis. Application of Celadrin cream and the oral use of Celadrin tablet/capsule is the best medication possible for immediate relief, free from side effects. Other safe and healthy options are Glucosamine Sulphate and Chondrotin Sulphate.